Cancer pain relief

SECOND EDITION

With a guide to opioid availability

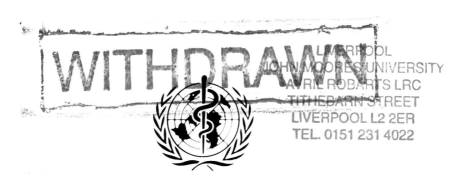

World Health Organization
Geneva
1996

WHO Library Cataloguing in Publication Data

Cancer pain relief : with a guide to opioid availability.
— 2nd ed.

1. Neoplasms – drug therapy   2. Pain – drug therapy
3. Palliative treatment   4. Narcotherapy

ISBN 92 4 154482 1   (NLM Classification: QZ 200)

The World Health Organization welcomes requests for permission to reproduce or translate its publications, in part or in full. Applications and enquiries should be addressed to the Office of Publications, World Health Organization, Geneva, Switzerland, which will be glad to provide the latest information on any changes made to the text, plans for new editions, and reprints and translations already available.

TYPESET IN HONG KONG
PRINTED IN SINGAPORE
95/10362 — Best-set/SNP — 14000

Contents

Preface

In most parts of the world, the majority of cancer patients present with advanced disease. For them, the only realistic treatment option is pain relief and palliative care. In 1986, the first edition of this publication proposed a method for relief of cancer pain, based on a small number of relatively inexpensive drugs, including morphine. Field-testing in several countries demonstrated the efficacy of the method in most cancer patients. The first edition has been translated into 22 languages and a total of over half a million copies have been sold, reflecting the growing awareness of the problem of cancer pain.

This second edition takes into account many of the advances in understanding and practice that have occurred since the mid-1980s. The groundwork for this revision was started in 1989, in the context of the meeting of a WHO Expert Committee on Cancer Pain Relief and Active Supportive Care.[1] Since then, each part of the book has been thoroughly revised and updated, and a section has been added on opioid availability.

It is important to note that cancer pain management should be undertaken as part of comprehensive palliative care.[2] Relief of other symptoms, and of psychological, social and spiritual problems, is paramount. Attempting to relieve pain without addressing the patient's non-physical concerns is likely to lead to frustration and failure.

---

[1] *Cancer pain relief and palliative care: report of a WHO Expert Committee.* Geneva, World Health Organization, 1990 (WHO Technical Report Series, No. 804).
[2] See, for example: Doyle D et al., eds. *Oxford textbook of palliative medicine.* Oxford, Oxford University Press, 1993.

Acknowledgements

The World Health Organization acknowledges the valuable contributions made to this book by the late Mr N. R. Donaldson, formerly Senior Consultant (Pharmacy), Drugs Directorate, Health Protection Branch, Department of Health and Welfare, Ottawa, Canada; Mr D. E. Joranson, Associate Director for Policy Studies, Pain Research Group, University of Wisconsin Medical School, Madison, WI, USA; Dr A. Sbanotto, Consultant Physician, Palliative Care Unit, European Institute of Oncology, Milan, Italy; Ms Noreen Teoh, formerly Technical Officer, Cancer and Palliative Care, WHO, Geneva, Switzerland; Dr R. Twycross, Director, WHO Collaborating Centre for Palliative Cancer Care, Oxford, England; and Professor V. Ventafridda, Director, WHO Collaborating Centre for Cancer Pain Relief, Milan, Italy.

PART I
Cancer pain relief

Introduction

The number of cancer patients in the world is increasing. Of the estimated nine million new cancer cases every year, more than half are in developing countries. The majority of these patients are incurable by the time their disease is diagnosed. Cancer mortality is expected to continue to rise in most regions of the world, mainly because of aging populations and increases in tobacco consumption.

Cancer patients need pain relief at all stages of their disease. Pain occurs in about one-third of patients receiving anticancer treatment. In these, pain relief measures and anticancer treatment go hand in hand. In patients with advanced disease, more than two-thirds experience pain, and the management of pain and other symptoms becomes the main aim of treatment.

The physiological basis of cancer pain includes a variety of mechanisms. The psychological aspects include anxiety, fear, depression and a sense of hopelessness. The aim of treatment is to relieve the pain to the patient's satisfaction, so that he or she can function effectively and eventually die free of pain.

Pain relief may be achieved by a variety of means (Table 1). Treatment must be tailored to the individual, with drug treatment and anaesthetic, neurosurgical, psychological and behavioural approaches geared to the patient's needs. This guide concentrates on drug treatment because there is sufficient knowledge and clinical experience to advocate its general implementation for all cancer patients who experience pain.

> Drug treatment is the mainstay of cancer pain management.

Field tests of these guidelines have shown that drugs are effective in a high percentage of patients, if used correctly — the right drug

Table I
Approaches to pain management in cancer patients

Psychological approaches:
understanding
companionship
cognitive behavioural therapies

Modification of pathological process:
radiotherapy
hormone therapy
chemotherapy
surgery

Drugs:
analgesics
antidepressants
anticonvulsants
anxiolytics
neuroleptics

Interruption of pain pathways:
local anaesthetics (lidocaine, bupivacaine)
neurolytic agents (alcohol, phenol, chlorocresol, cold, heat)
neurosurgery (e.g. cordotomy)

Modification of daily activities

Immobilization:
rest
cervical collar or corset
plastic splints or slings
orthopaedic surgery

in the right dose at the right time intervals. The drugs discussed here are commonly used for cancer pain management. Controlled studies have demonstrated the safety and efficacy of these drugs and of certain combinations of them. Not all the drugs are available in every country. In some circumstances, therefore, there will be a need to use alternative drugs.

A number of the terms used in this book are defined in Annex 1.

Causes of pain

Pain in patients with cancer may be:

- caused by the cancer itself (this is by far the most common);
- related to the cancer (e.g. muscle spasm, lymphoedema, constipation, bedsores);
- related to anticancer treatment (e.g. chronic postsurgical scar pain, chemotherapy-induced mucositis);
- caused by a concurrent disorder (e.g. spondylosis, osteoarthritis).

Many patients with advanced cancer have multiple pains from several of these categories.

The cancer itself causes pain through:

- extension into soft tissues;
- visceral involvement;
- bone involvement;
- nerve compression;
- nerve injury;
- raising intracranial pressure.

A series of specific pain syndromes unique to cancer (Table 2) have been described over the past 20 years (1). An awareness of these syndromes is necessary if the correct diagnosis is to be made. It is also important to consider the underlying neural mechanism (Table 3).

It is important to differentiate between burning pain associated with peripheral nerve injury (more common) and burning pain that is sympathetically maintained (less common). This can be difficult because the clinical features are not constant and some features

Table 2
Pain syndromes in patients with cancer[a]

Caused by cancer
Tumour involvement of bone:
   metastases to the cranial vault and base of skull
   metastases to vertebral body
      fracture of the odontoid process
      C7-T1 metastases
      L1 metastases
      sacral syndrome
Tumour involvement of viscera
Tumour involvement of nervous system:
   cranial neuralgia
   — trigeminal
   — glossopharyngeal
   peripheral nerves
   intercostal neuropathy
   brachial plexopathy
   lumbosacral plexopathy
   radiculopathy
   leptomeningeal metastases
   spinal cord compression
   intracranial metastases

Caused by anticancer treatment
Post-surgery:
   acute postoperative pain
   post-thoracotomy syndrome
   post-mastectomy syndrome
   post-neck-dissection syndrome
   phantom limb syndrome
Post-chemotherapy:
   oral mucositis
   bladder spasms
   aseptic necrosis of the femoral head
   steroid pseudorheumatism
   post-herpetic neuralgia
   peripheral neuropathy
Post-radiotherapy:
   oral mucositis
   oesophagitis
   skin burns
   radiation fibrosis of brachial and lumbar plexus
   radiation myelopathy
   radiation-induced second primary tumour

[a] Adapted from reference *1*.

Table 3
Classification of pain according to neural mechanism

Type of pain	Mechanism	Example
Nociceptive Visceral Somatic Muscle spasm	Stimulation of nerve endings	Hepatic capsule pain Bone pain Cramp
Neuropathic Nerve compression	Stimulation of nervi nervorum	
Nerve injury — peripheral[a]	Injury to peripheral nerve ("deafferentation pain")	Neuroma or nerve infiltration (e.g. brachial or lumbosacral plexus)
— central	Injury to central nervous system	Spinal cord compression or post- stroke pain
— mixed	Peripheral and central injury	Post-herpetic neuralgia
Sympathetically maintained[b]	Injury to sympathetic nerves	Some chronic post- surgical pains

[a] Characterized by superficial burning pain or stabbing pain with sensory loss in a neurodermatomal pattern.
[b] Characterized by superficial burning pain in an arterial pattern. Some nerve injury pains have a sympathetic component (e.g. Pancoast syndrome).

are common to both conditions. Peripheral nerve injury pain is neurodermatomal in distribution, whereas sympathetically maintained pain has an arterial distribution. Moreover, with sympathetically maintained pain, radiographs of the limb may show osteoporosis and an isotope bone scan may contain "hot spots", which can be mistaken for metastases.

If sympathetically maintained pain is suspected, a diagnostic sympathetic block with local anaesthetic should be undertaken if possible. This not only serves to confirm the diagnosis, but often gives relief that lasts longer than the duration of action of the local anaesthetic. If the pain returns, a neurolytic lumbar sympathetic block is worth considering for lower limb pain.

Evaluation of pain

Evaluation is a vital first step in cancer pain management. It demands an understanding of not only the physical problem, but also the psychological, social and spiritual components of the patient's suffering. It is best achieved by a team approach. The responsibility for evaluation lies primarily with the physician, but certain components may be undertaken by other health care workers.

The main steps in the evaluation of cancer pain are described below. Ignoring them leads, all too often, to misdiagnosis and inappropriate management.

1. Believe the patient's report of pain

2. Initiate discussions about pain
In the initial evaluation, the health worker should specifically ask the patient about pain, rather than relying on spontaneous comment. Sometimes a patient may be reluctant to admit to having pain, because of, for example, fear of injection or forced admission to hospital. If the patient is unable to describe the pain (e.g. an infant or a brain-damaged adult), the following may help to gauge the severity of the pain:

- observations by care-givers, e.g. parents;
- vocalizations, e.g. groaning;
- facial expressions, e.g. furrowed brow;
- changes in physiological responses, e.g. increase or decrease in blood pressure;
- response to a trial dose of analgesic.

3. Evaluate the severity of the pain

It is necessary to find out whether activity is limited by the pain, whether sleep is disturbed, and the degree of relief obtained with medication or pain-relief procedures, past and present. Formal pain scales can help, but they are not essential. With both children and adults, it is often helpful to offer a choice of descriptors (e.g. pressure, aching, burning, stabbing) and to ask the patient to relate the present pain to past pain, such as a toothache. Children under eight years of age cannot use the same scales or verbal processes as adults. Young children may be able to convey the intensity of their pain using a set of drawings of faces, ranging from smiling to crying, and selecting the face that best matches the pain. Alternatively, the child may be presented with four coins or pebbles and asked to indicate how many "pieces of hurt" he or she feels, with four objects indicating the worst pain. A similar approach can be used with patients who cannot read or write and where communication is difficult because of the lack of a common language.

4. Take a detailed history of the pain

A detailed history must be taken to discover the location and distribution of the pain, its quality and severity, whether it is continuous or intermittent, and what factors make it worse or better. Information should also be obtained about any weakness and sensory dysfunction. If possible, the history should be verified by speaking to a family member, who may provide information that the patient is unable or unwilling to give. This is particularly important with a patient who under-reports the severity of the pain and its impact on daily life. Information from the family member may provide the clue to the cause of the pain.

5. Evaluate the psychological state of the patient

Information about past illnesses, current level of anxiety and depression, suicidal thoughts, and the degree of functional incapacity helps to identify patients who may require more specific psychological support. Depression occurs in up to 25% of cancer patients. Other common psychiatric syndromes are also seen in patients with cancer pain. Detecting these is an important part of the total evaluation.

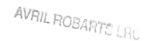

6. Perform a careful physical examination

A detailed history and a careful clinical examination may be all that is necessary to determine the cause of the pain so that appropriate treatment may begin.

7. Order and personally review any necessary investigations

Investigations should be reserved for cases where there is doubt about the cause of pain, or where a decision about further anticancer treatment depends on the precise localization of the disease. Although plain radiographs are a useful screening procedure, a negative result should not be used to overrule a clinical diagnosis. Plain radiographs are inadequate in areas of the body where bone shadows overlap, such as the base of the skull, C2, C7, T1 vertebral bodies, and the sacrum.

Although an isotope bone scan can demonstrate abnormalities in bone before changes appear on plain radiographs, it does not necessarily establish a diagnosis of bone metastasis. Osteoporosis, collapsed vertebral bodies, disuse atrophy, Paget disease and osteomyelitis can all give a positive bone scan. Likewise, a negative bone scan does not rule out bone metastasis. Further, in a previously irradiated site a bone scan is often negative even if active disease is present.

Computed tomography (CT) and magnetic resonance imaging (MRI) are the most useful diagnostic procedures in evaluating patients with cancer who are in pain. CT provides detailed visualization of bone and soft tissue and can identify early bony changes. MRI is particularly useful in evaluating vertebral body involvement, epidural spinal cord compression, and brain metastases. CT is also useful in directing needle placement for biopsy and for anaesthetic procedures such as coeliac plexus block.

Treatment with analgesic drugs often markedly improves a patient's ability to undergo necessary investigations. Since pain relief does not obscure the diagnosis, analgesics should not be withheld while the cause of the pain is being established.

8. Consider alternative methods of pain control

Although drug treatment is the mainstay of cancer pain management, alternative methods are of considerable benefit for some forms of cancer pain. For example, patients with painful bone metastases usually obtain considerable, or even complete, relief with palliative radiotherapy. If the pain is caused by a pathological fracture of the femur or humerus, orthopaedic pinning is often the treatment of choice.

9. Monitor the results of treatment

Continuing evaluation and treatment require a team approach and rely heavily on the observations of the health care worker who is delivering the care. The physician and other care-givers must establish regular and specific methods for sharing information about the effects of treatment so that, when necessary, changes in treatment can be made quickly. This entails continuity of care.

After evaluation, the physician should know whether the pain:

- is caused by the cancer or by another disorder;

- constitutes a specific cancer pain syndrome;

- is nociceptive, neuropathic or mixed nociceptive-neuropathic;

- is associated with a significant degree of psychological distress;

- is having a negative impact on the patient's family and/or care-givers.

Treatment strategy

Treatment should begin with a straightforward explanation to the patient of the causes of the pains. Many pains are best treated with a combination of drug and non-drug measures. Nevertheless, analgesics and a limited number of other drugs are the mainstay of cancer pain management (Table 4). Anticancer treatment and drug therapy for cancer pain can be given concurrently. Some pains respond well to a combination of a non-opioid and an opioid. With others, relief is obtained by combining a corticosteroid and an opioid. Neuropathic pains often show little response to non-opioid and opioid analgesics, but may be eased by tricyclic antidepressants and anticonvulsants. Recognizing that neuropathic pain is often resistant to opioids is important for optimal drug treatment.

Cancer patients often have many fears and anxieties, and may become depressed. Very anxious or deeply depressed patients may need an appropriate psychotropic drug in addition to an analgesic. If this fact is not appreciated, the pain may remain intractable.

Table 4
A basic drug list for cancer pain relief

Category	Basic drugs	Alternatives
Non-opioids	acetylsalicylic acid (ASA) paracetamol ibuprofen indometacin	choline magnesium trisalicylate diflunisal naproxen diclofenac
Opioids for mild to moderate pain[a]	codeine[b]	dihydrocodeine dextropropoxyphene standardized opium tramadol
Opioids for moderate to severe pain[a]	morphine	methadone hydromorphone oxycodone[c] levorphanol pethidine buprenorphine[c]
Opioid antagonist	naloxone	
Antidepressants[d]	amitriptyline	imipramine
Anticonvulsants[d]	carbamazepine	valproic acid
Corticosteroids[e]	prednisolone dexamethasone	prednisone betamethasone

[a] For practical purposes, the opioids are divided into those for mild to moderate pain and those for moderate to severe pain, principally on the grounds of common patterns of use.

[b] Codeine and some other opioids for mild to moderate pain are *not* scheduled drugs in most countries. This may make them more easily available.

[c] Buprenorphine is a partial agonist (i.e. it has a pharmacological ceiling). At low doses (0.2 mg every 8 hours), it is an alternative to codeine. At higher doses (up to 1 mg every 8 hours), it is equivalent to about 30 mg of oral morphine every 4 hours.

[d] Antidepressants and anticonvulsants are the drugs of choice for neuropathic pain.

[e] Of value in nerve compression and spinal cord compression pain; also for headache due to raised intracranial pressure. May be used as an alternative to, or in conjunction with, a nonsteroidal anti-inflammatory drug (NSAID) for bone pain. If used with an NSAID, there is an increased likelihood of adverse gastric effects and of fluid retention.

Use of analgesics

A relatively inexpensive yet effective method exists for relieving cancer pain in 70–90% of patients. A number of centres in different countries field-tested the method in the 1980s and demonstrated its efficacy. The method can be summarized in five phrases:

- "by mouth"
- "by the clock"
- "by the ladder"
- "for the individual"
- "attention to detail".

"By mouth"

If possible, analgesics should be given by mouth. Rectal suppositories are useful in patients with dysphagia, uncontrolled vomiting or gastrointestinal obstruction. Continuous subcutaneous infusion offers an alternative route in these situations. A number of mechanical and battery-powered portable infusion pumps are available.

"By the clock"

Analgesics should be given "by the clock", i.e. at fixed intervals of time. The dose of analgesic should be titrated against the patient's pain, i.e. gradually increased until the patient is comfortable. The next dose should be given before the effect of the previous one has fully worn off. In this way it is possible to relieve pain continuously.

Some patients need to take "rescue" doses for incident (intermittent) and breakthrough pain. Such doses, which should be

Fig. 1. The three-step analgesic ladder

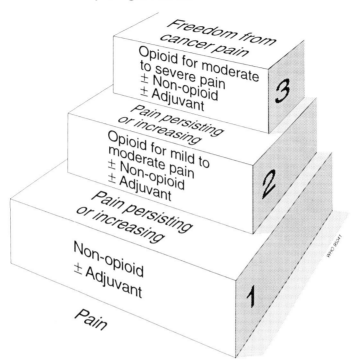

50–100% of the regular four-hourly dose, are in addition to the regular schedule.

"By the ladder"

The sequential use of the drugs is shown in Fig. 1. The first step is a non-opioid. If this does not relieve the pain, an opioid for mild to moderate pain should be added. When an opioid for mild to moderate pain in combination with a non-opioid fails to relieve the pain, an opioid for moderate to severe pain should be substituted. Only one drug from each of the groups should be used at the same time. Adjuvant drugs should be given for specific indications (see p. 32).

If a drug ceases to be effective, do not switch to an alternative drug of similar efficacy (e.g. from codeine to dextropropoxyphene), but prescribe a drug that is definitely stronger (e.g. morphine).

"For the individual"

There are no standard doses for opioid drugs. The "right" dose is the dose that relieves the patient's pain. The range for oral morphine, for example, is from as little as 5 mg to more than 1000 mg every four hours. Drugs used for mild to moderate pain have a dose limit in practice because of formulation (e.g. combined with ASA or paracetamol, which are toxic at high doses) or because of a disproportionate increase in adverse effects at higher doses (e.g. codeine).

"Attention to detail"

Emphasize the need for regular administration of pain-relief drugs. Oral morphine should be administered every four hours. The first and last doses of the day should be linked to the patient's waking time and bedtime. The best additional times during the day are generally 10:00, 14:00 and 18:00. With this schedule, there is a balance between duration of analgesic effect and severity of adverse effects.

Ideally, the patient's drug regimen should be **written out in full** for the patient and his or her family to work from, including names of drugs, reason for use (e.g. "for pain", "for bowels"), dose (number of ml, number of tablets) and number of times per day. The patient should be warned about possible adverse effects.

Choice of analgesic

Non-opioid analgesics

The non-opioid analgesics include acetylsalicylic acid (ASA), other nonsteroidal anti-inflammatory drugs (NSAIDs) and paracetamol. ASA, paracetamol, ibuprofen and indometacin are all included in the *Model list of essential drugs* (2). In most countries, a number of NSAIDs are available, and the choice will depend on factors such as local availability and cost.

NSAIDs, including ASA, are particularly important in the treatment of pain caused by bone metastases. There is often a high local concentration of prostaglandins in the affected bone produced by the tumour cells, and NSAIDs act partly by blocking prostaglandin biosynthesis. Patients with bone pain who are intolerant of ASA should be given an alternative NSAID (Table 4).

The non-opioids are also particularly helpful for pain caused by soft tissue and muscle infiltration. Drugs in this group display a "ceiling" effect, i.e. increasing the dose above a given level does not provide further relief. If pain is not adequately relieved by a non-opioid, an opioid should be added.

Use of non-opioid analgesics

Dose recommendations for non-opioid analgesics are contained in Table 5.

To minimize the risk of allergic phenomena, ask the patient beforehand whether he or she can tolerate ASA and ASA-like compounds. If troublesome adverse effects occur, change to an alternative non-opioid. If the adverse effects persist, change to an opioid. For patients with impaired platelet function, use either paracetamol or non-acetylated salicylate, e.g. choline magnesium trisalicylate or diflunisal. Doses of diflunisal in excess of 1 g a day may, however, adversely affect platelet function.

Table 5
Non-opioid drugs for relief of cancer pain

Drug	Standard dose	Adverse effects
Acetylsalicylic acid (ASA)	500–600 mg every 4–6 hours	Gastric irritation — dyspepsia and faecal blood loss
	Adverse gastric effects may be reduced if ASA is taken with milk, after food, or with antacids. The administration of more than 4 g/day is likely to lead to toxic effects such as tinnitus, deafness and other symptoms of salicylism.	
	Some cytotoxic drugs (e.g. methotrexate) are highly protein-bound and will be partly displaced by salicylates. This will result in increased toxicity unless the dose is adjusted accordingly.	
	Note: May be given as a suppository.	
Paracetamol	650–1000 mg every 4–6 hours	Liver and renal toxicity
	Use with caution in patients with liver damage. The total dose per day should not exceed 6 g.	
	Note: May be given as a suppository.	
Ibuprofen	400 mg every 4–6 hours	Less likelihood of adverse gastrointestinal effects
	Increasing relief is obtained with doses up to 3 g per day.	
Indometacin	25 mg every 6 hours	Greater likelihood of adverse gastrointestinal effects
	Maximum recommended daily dose is 200 mg.	
	Note: May be given as a suppository.	

Hypersensitivity occurs occasionally as an idiosyncratic reaction. This syndrome may develop within minutes of drug ingestion. Manifestations range from vasomotor rhinitis with profuse watery secretion, angioneurotic oedema, urticaria and bronchial asthma to laryngeal oedema and bronchoconstriction, hypotension, shock, loss of consciousness and complete vasomotor collapse. This reaction may occur in response to even small amounts of ASA or other NSAIDs.

> When a non-opioid drug no longer adequately controls the pain,
> an opioid analgesic should be added.

Opioid analgesics

For practical purposes, opioid analgesics can be divided into those used for **mild to moderate pain** and those used for **moderate to severe pain**. This distinction is arbitrary; it is based on the existence of the ceiling effect and on the manner in which these drugs are usually prescribed.

Opioid analgesics given by mouth provide effective pain relief for most patients and are simple to administer. The safe and rational use of opioid analgesics requires an understanding of their clinical pharmacology.

The use of opioid analgesics is associated with the development of physical dependence and tolerance. These are normal pharmacological responses to the continuing use of these drugs. Physical dependence is characterized by withdrawal symptoms if treatment is stopped abruptly or if an antagonist is injected. Tolerance is characterized by decreased efficacy and duration of action of the drug with repeated administration, requiring an increased dose to maintain the analgesic effect. In practice, physical dependence and tolerance do not prevent the effective use of these drugs. Patients with stable disease often remain on a stable dose for weeks or months.

Psychological dependence, or "drug dependence" (3), is a behavioural pattern characterized by craving for the drug and an overwhelming preoccupation with obtaining it. Undue anxiety about psychological dependence has caused physicians and patients to use inadequate doses of opioids. Wide clinical experience has shown that psychological dependence does not occur in cancer patients as a result of receiving opioids for relief of pain. This is true of both children and adults.

It should be emphasized that the use of opioids can be stopped if the cause of pain is dealt with by anticancer treatment (e.g. radiotherapy or chemotherapy). To avoid withdrawal symptoms, the dose should be decreased gradually. After an abrupt reduction in pain (e.g. after a nerve block or neuroablative procedure), the dose should be reduced to 25% of the original dose. If the procedure has been successful, the dose can be reduced further every 2–3 days, and stopped completely if the pain does not recur. In this way, withdrawal symptoms are avoided.

Several factors must be considered if opioids are to be used effectively. These include:

- previous opioid exposure;
- severity and nature of the pain;
- age of the patient;
- extent of cancer, particularly hepatic and renal involvement;
- concurrent disease.

Because the response of each patient varies, it is necessary to select the most appropriate drug and administer it in the dose that best suits the individual. There is no standard recommended dose. Low starting doses should be used in elderly people, who may have an increased response because of changes in the pharmacokinetics of opioids. Starting doses for children should be based on body weight.

Most opioid analgesics are metabolized primarily in the liver, and their elimination is therefore dependent on liver function. Liver disease is not, however, a contraindication to the use of opioids. In patients with liver cirrhosis, oral systemic bioavailability (the fraction of an oral dose reaching the systemic circulation) has been shown to be increased for dextropropoxyphene and pethidine (Table 6). Concomitantly, the rate of clearance of the drug from the blood is decreased and the intensity and duration of action of the drug are increased. This may lead to accentuation of drug effects at comparatively low doses.

The metabolites of most drugs are excreted by the kidneys. Renal dysfunction can therefore lead to an accumulation of metabolites (Table 6). This is particularly relevant in the case of morphine, because morphine-6-glucuronide (M6G) is an active metabolite.

Table 6
Disease-induced alterations in opioid pharmacokinetics[a]

Disease	Opioid	Effect
Cirrhosis	Dextropropoxyphene	Increased bioavailability, decreased clearance
	Pethidine	Increased bioavailability, decreased clearance
Renal failure	Dihydrocodeine	Decreased clearance
	Dextropropoxyphene	Increased norpropoxyphene (a toxic metabolite)
	Morphine	Increased morphine-6-glucuronide (an active metabolite)
	Pethidine	Increased norpethidine (a toxic metabolite)

[a] Adapted from reference *4*.

The plasma half-life of M6G varies between 2.5 and 7.5 hours, and central depression, i.e. sedation and respiratory depression, will result unless the dose of morphine is reduced. Pethidine is metabolized to norpethidine, which has a normal half-life of 12–16 hours. Norpethidine causes myoclonus and seizures at high concentrations. Pethidine should therefore not be used in patients with renal dysfunction, and morphine should be used with caution.

Some liver and kidney diseases are associated with low albumin levels. This may decrease plasma-protein binding and hence increase the response to opioids. Severe malnutrition may alter the distribution and availability of these drugs in the body, thereby modifying their effects. The lack of data on use of opioids in malnourished patients means that caution is necessary. Malnutrition is not, however, a contraindication for opioid use.

A longer plasma half-life in the newborn may explain the prolonged duration of action of morphine in this group. In infants older than one month, however, the morphine metabolism is the same as or more rapid than in adults.

Use of opioid analgesics

Two opioids — codeine and morphine — are contained in the *Model list of essential drugs* (2), while pethidine is on the complementary list. Other opioids are available in many countries. Although pethidine is of value in the treatment of acute severe pain, it has a number of disadvantages when used regularly in cancer patients. It should not be used if alternatives are available.

Codeine by mouth

Codeine may be given by mouth in doses of 30–120 mg every four hours. Above this dose, adverse effects tend to increase disproportionately to pain relief. The adverse effects of codeine are essentially those common to all opioids (see page 27).

Morphine by mouth

Morphine can be given as:

- a simple aqueous solution of the sulfate or hydrochloride salt every four hours (an antimicrobial preservative may be added);
- tablets, every 4 hours;
- slow-release tablets, every 12 hours.

The effective analgesic dose of morphine varies considerably and ranges from as little as 5 mg to more than 1000 mg every four hours. In most patients, pain is controlled with doses of 10–30 mg every four hours. The effective dose varies partly because of individual variations in systemic bioavailability. **The correct dose is the dose that works.** The drug must be given "by the clock" and not merely when the patient complains of pain. The use of morphine should be dictated by intensity of pain, not by life expectancy.

If the patient has a sudden attack of severe pain, a rescue dose of morphine should be given promptly and repeated after one hour if necessary. After the pain has been relieved, the regular dose should be reviewed, and increased if necessary.

Slow-release morphine tablets are available in some countries in strengths varying from 10 mg to 200 mg. These tablets usually need be given only every 12 hours.

Other opioid analgesics

In most patients requiring an opioid for moderate to severe pain, morphine is both efficacious and acceptable, and is the drug of choice. If a patient appears to be intolerant to morphine, an alternative should be tried.

Standardized opium

Standardized opium is essentially dilute morphine. The morphine content varies but is usually 10% of the weight of opium powder. In some countries, opium is combined with ASA in a fixed-dose tablet.

Tramadol

Tramadol is a synthetic, centrally acting analgesic, with both opioid and non-opioid properties. It is promptly absorbed by the gastrointestinal tract, resulting in 70% bioavailability. Although its potency relative to orally administered codeine and morphine is still being debated, it seems to be about twice as potent as codeine and one-fifth as potent as morphine. When administered parenterally, tramadol has about one-tenth the potency of morphine. Biotransformation produces an active metabolite, which is 2–4 times more potent than tramadol, and has a plasma half-life of about 6 hours. The usual oral dose is 50–100 mg, every 4–6 hours. Tramadol causes less constipation and respiratory depression than other opioids at equianalgesic doses. Because of its low dependence liability, it is not a controlled drug.

Hydromorphone

When given by mouth hydromorphone is about eight times more potent than morphine, but only six times more potent by injection. The duration of action is 3–4 hours. The usual starting dose is 1–2 mg by mouth or 1 mg by subcutaneous injection. By injection, most patients need $\frac{1}{3}$ to $\frac{1}{2}$ of the previously satisfactory oral dose.

Methadone

Methadone is a synthetic opioid analgesic with effects generally similar to those of morphine. Given orally, it is about half as effective as when given by subcutaneous injection. Its plasma half-life varies from about 8 to 80 hours. Steady-state levels may be achieved after 7–14 days. This must be taken into account, otherwise problems are likely to occur as a result of accumulation, especially in people who are debilitated or elderly. Its effective analgesic dose range is the same as that of morphine. It produces analgesia lasting 6–12 hours.

Greater care needs to be exercised when using methadone, as compared with morphine, particularly at first when the patient's response to it is not fully known. Extra care should be taken if psychotropic drugs are being administered concurrently.

Rifampicin, an antituberculous antibiotic, speeds up the metabolism of methadone and may, on occasion, precipitate withdrawal symptoms.

Levorphanol

Levorphanol is about five times more potent than morphine, and provides relief for about six hours. Like methadone, it may accumulate in the blood and may produce sedation with repeated doses. The normal starting dose is 2 mg four times a day by mouth. If the drug is given by injection, the dose should be halved.

Pethidine

Pethidine is a synthetic opioid analgesic. Its effects are generally similar to those of morphine. It also has anticholinergic properties. It is not as effective as morphine in relieving severe pain, but in higher doses it is considerably more effective than codeine. It is generally shorter-acting than morphine, with useful analgesia lasting up to three hours.

Pethidine is *not* a complete alternative to morphine. It may need to be given every three hours in patients with severe cancer pain because of its shorter duration of action. Doses of pethidine and morphine that have equivalent analgesic effects also produce a similar incidence of adverse effects.

With pethidine, the incidence of adverse central nervous system (CNS) effects (tremor, twitching, agitation and convulsions) increases considerably at doses above 100 mg every three hours. Pethidine should not be given to patients:

- with impaired renal function, because of the increased likelihood of adverse central nevous system effects

- who are taking monoamine oxidase inhibitors because of the likelihood of a hypertensive or hypotensive crisis.

Phenobarbital and chlorpromazine increase the toxicity of pethidine.

Oxycodone

Oxycodone is a synthetic derivative of thebaine, and is structurally related to codeine. Oxycodone hydrochloride has good oral bioavailability (approximately 50–70%) and seems to be as potent as morphine. The analgesic effect lasts from 3 to 5 hours. The existence of a limiting dose is a subject of debate. As the pectinate, oxycodone can be administered rectally, giving a slightly longer duration of analgesia. Side-effects are similar to those of morphine.

Buprenorphine

Buprenorphine is a partial agonist; it produces morphine-like effects, but has a ceiling of 3–5 mg per day. It is not, therefore, a complete alternative to morphine. If given at the same time as morphine or another strong opioid in high doses, there is a possibility of a *decreased* analgesic effect, because of displacement of the full agonist (morphine) from opioid receptors by the partial agonist (buprenorphine).

The onset of action occurs about 30 minutes after administration, and the peak effect is seen after three hours. The duration of useful effect is 6–9 hours. Most patients are satisfactorily controlled on an eight-hour regimen. The drug is taken sublingually or parenterally (0.4 mg sublingually is equivalent to 0.3 mg by injection). If buprenorphine is swallowed, the effect is much reduced by "first-pass" hepatic metabolism.

Table 7
Oral opioids for moderate to severe pain: typical starting doses

Opioid	Starting dose (mg)
morphine	10–15
hydromorphone	1–2
oxycodone	5–15
methadone	5–10
levorphanol	1–2
pethidine	50–100

Sublingual buprenorphine is about 60 times more potent than orally administered morphine, i.e. 0.2 mg sublingually every 8 hours is equivalent to 6 mg of morphine given orally every 4 hours. Patients whose pain is no longer controlled by buprenorphine should be given oral morphine sulfate instead. The starting daily dose of morphine in this case should be 100 times the previously administered total daily dose of buprenorphine. This dose should be converted into a convenient four-hourly morphine regimen.

Choice of starting dose
The initial dose of an opioid for moderate to severe pain depends mainly on the patient's previous medication. For those who have previously received 60–100 mg of codeine by mouth, a starting dose of 10–15 mg of morphine is usually adequate (Table 7).

If the patient is very somnolent after the first dose and is free of pain, the second dose should be 50% lower. If, after 24 hours on the medication, pain relief is inadequate, the starting dose should be increased. The amount of additional medication needed will serve as a guide to the patient's requirements. A typical increment is 50%, though it may be more initially. Meanwhile, rescue doses can be given. The patient must be re-evaluated after 24 and 72 hours, preferably by the physician.

Night doses
The drug should be given through the night, or in a larger dose at bedtime to sustain the plasma level of the drug within the effective range. With a double dose of morphine at bedtime, many patients do not need a further dose until morning. A double dose is not

necessary with slow-release preparations, or with longer-acting drugs such as methadone and buprenorphine.

Adverse effects
Constipation is the most common adverse effect. The use of laxatives is discussed under adjuvant drugs (see p. 33).

Nausea and vomiting occur in over 50% of cancer patients receiving opioids for moderate to severe pain. The use of antiemetics is discussed under adjuvant drugs (see p. 32).

Drowsiness and confusion. The patient should be warned about initial drowsiness. Usually this will clear up after 3–5 days on a constant dose. The same is true of confusion, which occurs principally in elderly patients. However, if the patient is heavily sedated or markedly confused, it may be necessary to reduce the dose and re-titrate more slowly.

A few patients experience continuing marked sedation. Except in patients who are close to death, the most common cause of continuing sedation is the concurrent use of psychotropic drugs (anxiolytics and neuroleptics). Reducing the dose of the psychotropic drug or changing to a less sedative alternative (e.g. from chlorpromazine to haloperidol) normally leads to improvement. Occasionally a psychostimulant (e.g. methylphenidate) may help. Sometimes, changing to an alternative opioid is helpful (e.g. from morphine to oxycodone, hydromorphone, levorphanol or methadone). If all else fails and the patient's pain is poorly relieved, the spinal route of administration should be considered.

Respiratory depression. Pain is the physiological antagonist to the central depressant effects of opioids. Clinically important respiratory depression is rare in cancer patients because the dose of the opioid is balanced by the underlying pain. Patients who become very sedated by the medication may, however, develop respiratory depression. This may occur during the initial titration or because of metabolic dysfunction. Respiratory depression can be reversed immediately by the intravenous administration of 0.2–0.4 mg of naloxone, an opioid antagonist. In patients who are taking drugs with a long plasma half-life, such as methadone or levorphanol, it may be necessary to administer naloxone every 2–3 hours. Very large doses of naloxone, up to 4 mg, may be necessary to reverse respiratory depression caused by buprenorphine.

Rare effects. Occasionally, a patient may experience opioid-induced psychotic symptoms or symptoms relating to histamine release (pruritus, bronchoconstriction). These patients should be changed to an alternative strong opioid analgesic (see Table 4).

Alternative routes for administration of morphine and other opioids
Most patients are able to take morphine and other opioids by mouth. Towards the end of life, however, it is often necessary to make use of alternative routes because of dysphagia.

Rectal administration
Morphine may be given per rectum; this is as effective as by mouth. It is contraindicated in immunosuppressed neutropenic patients because minor rectal trauma may result in local cellulitis.

In some countries, morphine suppositories are available in strengths ranging from 10 mg to 60 mg. When suppositories are not available, morphine can be given by rectal enema, in 10–20 ml of water. Slow-release tablets can also be given by this route. Other opioids can also be given per rectum. This route should not be used in patients with diarrhoea or faecal incontinence.

Subcutaneous administration
In patients unable to take oral or rectal morphine, the subcutaneous route should be used. Repeated injections should be avoided if possible because most patients find them unpleasant. Continuous subcutaneous infusion using a portable syringe driver is preferable. If a syringe driver is not available, a butterfly cannula can be left *in situ* and morphine injected intermittently. By injection, most patients need one-third to one-half of the previously satisfactory oral dose. Buprenorphine, hydromorphone and levorphanol can also be given subcutaneously.

Intramuscular administration
If given by injection, pethidine should be given intramuscularly because it causes tissue irritation.

Intravenous administration

Opioids may be given intravenously by either bolus injection or continuous infusion.

> The dose of morphine or other opioid is the same whether given subcutaneously, intramuscularly or intravenously.

Spinal administration

The epidural and intrathecal routes provide pain relief with few adverse effects. These routes are important in patients who experience severe adverse effects or who have pain that is poorly responsive to opioids. As spinal administration requires special expertise and equipment for catheter placement, these routes will not be practicable in many settings.

If a patient has developed physical dependence on opioids administered by more conventional routes, withdrawal symptoms may occur when spinal administration is started. These may be avoided by continuing to give one-quarter of the dose by the former route, reducing the amount progressively over several days.

Transdermal administration

Certain drugs, with an adequate oil/water partition coefficient, low relative molecular mass and sufficient potency, can be administered transdermally. Fentanyl citrate has recently been proposed for administration by this route. Application of fentanyl patches produces a slow increase in plasma levels of the drug: peak plasma concentrations are achieved after 12–24 hours and a depot remains in the skin for 24 hours after the patch is removed. Rescue medication may be necessary during the first 24 hours. Doses vary from 75 µg/hour to 350 µg/hour. Compliance of patients is generally very good, but the cost of this method and its current limited availability restrict its use.

Drugs for neuropathic pain

As with nociceptive pain, drug treatment is the mainstay of man-

29

agement for neuropathic pain. One or more of the following groups of drugs may help:

- tricyclic antidepressants;
- anticonvulsants;
- local anaesthetic congeners (class I anti-arrhythmics).

Patients with neuropathic pain may derive benefit from opioids, particularly in cases of nerve compression. However, nerve compression pain may respond only if a corticosteroid is added. Mixed nociceptive and neuropathic pain will also benefit from morphine. Superficial burning pain and spontaneous stabbing pain associated with nerve injury often responds best to a tricyclic antidepressant or an anticonvulsant.

Tricyclic antidepressants

Amitriptyline and imipramine are both widely available. Alternative preparations are available in many countries and may be more suitable for some patients. Nortriptyline does not have a sedative effect; desipramine is relatively nonsedative and has minimal anticholinergic effects.

The starting dose will depend on the patient's age, weight, previous use of such drugs and concurrent medication. A dose as low as 10 mg may be appropriate for some patients, but most can take 25–50 mg. The dose should be increased to 30–50 mg as rapidly as can be tolerated in terms of sedation, postural hypotension and dry mouth. After that, increments should be made on a weekly basis until the pain is relieved or adverse effects preclude further escalation. Except with nortriptyline, the total daily dose should be given at bedtime, because most tricyclic antidepressants have a sedative effect. An analgesic effect is seen in many patients after a few days on doses of 50–100 mg. The pain is not, however, always completely relieved.

In children, the recommended starting dose is 0.5 mg/kg of body weight, increasing to 1 mg/kg if necessary.

Anticonvulsants

Extensive clinical experience supports the use of anticonvulsants such as carbamazepine and valproic acid in the treatment of nerve injury pain, particularly stabbing pain.

Carbamazepine

The starting dose of carbamazepine is 100 mg twice daily. This can be increased slowly, at a rate of 200 mg every few days. Carbamazepine causes enzyme autoinduction, thereby enhancing its own metabolism. This is one reason why initial adverse effects (e.g. drowsiness, ataxia) improve with time. Carbamazepine occasionally causes leukopenia.

This drug should not be used in children under six years of age. In older children, start by giving 100 mg/day (2–3 mg/kg of body weight), and increase in stages to 500 mg/day if necessary. Carbamazepine may exacerbate pre-existing chemotherapy-induced suppression of bone marrow.

Valproic acid

Valproic acid has a long plasma half-life and is sedative. It may conveniently be given as a single dose at bedtime, at a starting dose of 500 mg, or 200 mg for elderly patients. The dose may be increased by 200 mg, if necessary, every 3–4 days to a maximum of 1–1.5 g. As the drug accumulates in the body, the dose may subsequently have to be reduced.

Valproic acid should not be used in children under two years of age because of the danger of hepatotoxicity, which may be fatal.

Local anaesthetic congeners

Lidocaine given intravenously and oral flecainide and mexiletine are membrane-stabilizing drugs, and often relieve neuropathic pain. Flecainide is given in a dose of 50–200 mg twice a day and mexiletine 150 mg 2–4 times a day. Because anti-arrhythmics can become pro-arrhythmic under certain circumstances, it is generally advised *not* to administer flecainide or mexiletine concurrently with a tricyclic antidepressant.

Table 8
Adjuvant drugs

	Analgesic effect	Anti-depressant effect	Anxiolytic effect	Muscle relaxant	Antiemetic effect
Corticosteroids	+[a]				+
Psychotropic drugs:					
diazepam			+	+	
hydroxyzine	+[b]		+		+
haloperidol			+		+
prochlorperazine			+		+
chlorpromazine			+		+
amitriptyline	+[c]	+	+		

[a] Used in nerve compression, spinal cord compression and raised intracranial pressure.
[b] An analgesic effect has been reported when 100 mg is given by injection with morphine.
[c] Used as the primary analgesic for neuropathic pain.

Adjuvant drugs

Adjuvant drugs (Table 8) may be necessary for one of three reasons:

- to treat the adverse effects of analgesics (e.g. antiemetics and laxatives);
- to enhance pain relief (e.g. a corticosteroid in nerve compression pain);
- to treat concomitant psychological disturbances such as insomnia, anxiety and depression (e.g. night sedatives, anxiolytics and antidepressants).

Antiemetics

If the patient has nausea when first given an opioid, a neuroleptic antiemetic should be prescribed concurrently, e.g. haloperidol, 1–2 mg once a day, increasing to a maximum of 5 mg. Prochlorperazine, 5 mg every 8 hours, increasing to a maximum of 10 mg every 4 hours, is a useful alternative.

A small number of patients receiving morphine develop nausea and vomiting that are unresponsive to neuroleptics, possibly as a result of drug-induced delayed gastric emptying. Metoclopramide (10 mg every 8 hours, increasing to a maximum of 20 mg every 4 hours) should be substituted for the neuroleptic. If the vomiting persists, consider changing to a continuous subcutaneous infusion of morphine with metoclopramide, 60 mg per day, for several days.

If the patient vomits several times a day, the antiemetic will need to be given by injection, initially for two days. In patients with inoperable bowel obstruction, an antihistaminic antiemetic, such as cyclizine or dimenhydrinate can be given. To reduce gastrointestinal secretions, an atropine-like drug, such as hyoscine butylbromide, may be necessary.

Laxatives

As a general rule, a laxative should be prescribed when an opioid is started. The dose of laxative needed varies considerably from patient to patient. It may take 1–2 weeks to find the right dose. Between one-third and one-half of the patients need laxative suppositories or enemas in addition to an oral laxative, particularly at first.

For most patients, the regular use of a peristaltic stimulant, such as senna, counteracts opioid-induced constipation. The dose has to be titrated for each patient until a satisfactory result is achieved. Two tablets of standardized senna twice a day is a typical starting-dose for patients receiving opioids, increasing to two tablets every four hours if necessary. Some patients may require a faecal softener, e.g. docusate, 200 mg, 2–3 times daily. If the patient is severely constipated when an opioid is first prescribed, the use of laxative suppositories (e.g. bisacodyl) or an enema is an important first step.

Corticosteroids

There is a wide range of indications for using corticosteroids in patients with advanced cancer (Table 9). Corticosteroids are useful for relieving pain associated with nerve compression or spinal cord compression, and headache from raised intracranial pressure.

Table 9
Possible indications for corticosteroids in advanced cancer[a]

General uses	Specific indications for use
To improve appetite	Spinal cord compression
To enhance sense of well-being	Nerve compression
To improve strength	Dyspnoea:
Hormone therapy:	— pneumonitis (after radiotherapy)
— replacement	— carcinomatous lymphangitis
— anticancer	— tracheal compression/stridor
To relieve pain caused by:	Superior vena caval obstruction
— raised intracranial	Pericardial effusion
pressure	Haemoptysis
— nerve compression	Obstruction of hollow viscus:
— spinal cord compression	— bronchus
— metastatic arthralgia	— ureter
— bone metastasis	— intestine
	Hypercalcaemia (in lymphoma, myeloma)
	Radiation-induced inflammation
	Leukoerythroblastic anaemia
	Rectal discharge (give per rectum)
	Sweating

[a] Source: reference 5.

Both prednisolone and dexamethasone are effective; 1 mg of dexamethasone is equivalent to 7 mg of prednisolone.

The dose will depend on the clinical situation. For nerve compression pain, 20–40 mg of prednisolone or 4–6 mg of dexamethasone per day should be prescribed, reducing step by step to a maintenance dose after one week. The maintenance dose will depend on the amount needed to relieve pain, but could be as low as 15 mg of prednisolone or 2 mg of dexamethasone. Occasionally, a higher dose may be necessary to achieve significant benefit.

In patients with raised intracranial pressure, an initial daily dose of 8–16 mg of dexamethasone is appropriate. It may be possible to begin to reduce this to a maintenance dose after one week. With spinal cord compression, even higher doses have been used in some centres — up to 100 mg per day initially, reducing to 16 mg during radiation therapy.

Adverse effects include oedema, dyspeptic symptoms and, occasionally, gastrointestinal bleeding. Proximal myopathy, agitation, hypomania and opportunistic infections may also occur. The incidence of adverse gastrointestinal effects is increased if corticosteroids are used in conjunction with NSAIDs.

Psychotropic drugs

Many cancer patients with pain need a psychotropic drug (Table 8). For some, it may be the best analgesic for their pain, e.g. a tricyclic antidepressant for nerve injury pain. For others, it may be an antiemetic, e.g. haloperidol for opioid-induced vomiting. In others, an anxiolytic, such as diazepam, may be necessary. Diazepam is also useful in patients with muscle spasm or myofascial trigger point pain. Some patients need a night sedative and others need an antidepressant for identifiable depression.

The concurrent use of two drugs that act on the central nervous system (e.g. morphine plus a psychotropic drug, or two psychotropic drugs together) is likely to produce a greater sedative effect in ill and malnourished cancer patients than in others. In patients with cancer pain, the starting dose of a psychotropic drug may need to be less than that used for physically healthy patients.

Summary

1. Cancer pain can, and should, be treated.

2. Evaluation and treatment of cancer pain are best achieved by a team approach.

3. The first steps are to take a detailed history, and to examine the patient carefully, to determine if the pain is:

   - caused by the cancer, related to the cancer, caused by anticancer treatment or caused by another disorder;

   - part of a specific syndrome;

   - nociceptive, neuropathic, or mixed nociceptive and neuropathic.

4. Treatment begins with an explanation and combines physical and psychological approaches, using both non-drug and drug treatments.

5. It is useful to have a sequence of specific aims, such as:

   - to increase the hours of pain-free sleep;

   - to relieve the pain when the patient is at rest;

   - to relieve pain when the patient is standing or active.

6. Drugs alone usually give adequate relief from pain caused by cancer, provided that the right drug is administered in the right dose at the right time intervals.

7. "By mouth": the oral route is the preferred route for analgesics, including morphine.

8. "By the clock": for persistent pain, drugs should be taken at regular time intervals and not "as needed".

36

9. "By the ladder":

- Unless the patient is in severe pain, begin by prescribing a non-opioid drug and adjust the dose, if necessary, to the maximum recommended dose.

- If or when the non-opioid no longer adequately relieves the pain, an opioid drug should be prescribed **in addition to the non-opioid.**

- If or when an opioid for mild to moderate pain (e.g. codeine) no longer adequately relieves the pain, it should be replaced by an opioid for moderate to severe pain (e.g. morphine).

10. "For the individual": the right dose of an analgesic is the dose that relieves the pain. The dose of oral morphine may range from as little as 5 mg to more than 1000 mg.

11. Adjuvant drugs should be prescribed as indicated.

12. For neuropathic pain, a tricyclic antidepressant or an anticonvulsant is the analgesic of choice.

13. "Attention to detail": it is essential to monitor the patient's response to the treatment to ensure that the patient obtains maximum benefit with as few adverse effects as possible.

PART 2
Opioid availability

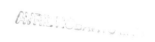

Introduction

Background

This part explains the system by which morphine and other opioids are made available to patients who need them. It is intended for use by both drug regulators and health care workers and to promote communication between the two groups. Opioid availability is discussed in the context of the problem of cancer pain and international efforts to address it. A number of the terms used in what follows are defined in Annex 1.

The text has been reviewed by the International Narcotics Control Board (INCB), the body responsible for administering the Single Convention on Narcotic Drugs (6), the treaty that governs opioid availability in the world. National drug regulatory authorities in ten countries have also commented on the text.

New knowledge, new hope

Research in management of cancer pain has produced new knowledge about pain and how opioids act in the body in relation to pain. Traditionally, the opioid analgesics have been used to manage acute pain. Long-term use of opioids has been discouraged because of the risk of tolerance or physical or psychological dependence. Studies have shown that, while physical dependence and tolerance do occur in patients who take opioids over a long period, psychological dependence is extremely rare. Consequently, the risk of such dependence should not be a factor in deciding whether to use opioids to treat the cancer patient with pain.

Studies have also shown that morphine and some other opioids do not have a "ceiling effect". Morphine can be safely administered in increasing amounts until the pain is relieved without producing an "overdose", as long as the side-effects are tolerated. There is no standard dose of morphine; the correct dose is the one that relieves the pain. This dose may vary from patient to patient; a few patients with severe pain may require several thousand milligrams of oral morphine daily to relieve pain.

In general, studies on the use of opioids to treat pain in cancer patients indicate that public and professional expectations about relief from cancer pain should be much higher than they are at present.

Impediments to cancer pain relief

There are many reasons why cancer pain is not adequately treated at present (7), including:

- absence of national policies on cancer pain relief and palliative care;
- lack of awareness on the part of health care workers, policy-makers, administrators and the public that most cancer pain can be relieved;
- shortage of financial resources and limitations of health care delivery systems and personnel;
- concern that medical use of opioids will produce psychological dependence and drug abuse;
- legal restrictions on the use and availability of opioid analgesics.

The WHO strategy

To respond to these issues, WHO advocates a strategy with the following key components (Fig. 2):

- national or state policies that support cancer pain relief through government endorsement of education and drug availability;
- educational programmes for the public, health care personnel, regulators, etc.;
- modification of laws and regulations to improve the availability of drugs, especially the opioid analgesics.

Fig. 2. Foundation measures for implementing cancer pain relief programmes

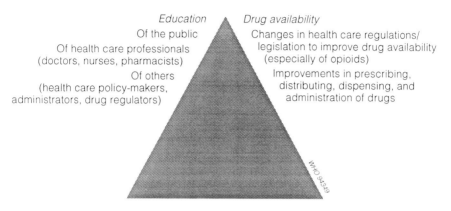

Education
Of the public
Of health care professionals
(doctors, nurses, pharmacists)
Of others
(health care policy-makers,
administrators, drug regulators)

Drug availability
Changes in health care regulations/
legislation to improve drug availability
(especially of opioids)
Improvements in prescribing,
distributing, dispensing, and
administration of drugs

Government policy
National or state policy emphasizing the need to alleviate
chronic cancer pain

These foundation measures are important if existing knowledge is to be implemented rationally. They cost very little but can have a significant effect (*14*).

Difficulties in obtaining opioids

Fig. 3 shows the global consumption of morphine according to population density. It can be seen that morphine consumption varies greatly from country to country. Consumption figures do not completely indicate the extent to which opioids are used for treatment of moderate to severe cancer pain; however, they provide probably the best single indicator available.

WHO monitors morphine consumption in individual countries as an index of improvements in pain management. Global morphine consumption was relatively stable until 1984, when WHO began to emphasize the need to use morphine in the treatment of cancer pain. From 1984 to 1992, global consumption of morphine more than tripled.

Many countries have fundamental difficulties in obtaining and distributing drugs for any type of illness. In these countries, the

Fig. 3. Morphine consumption, in mg per person, 1984 and 1992

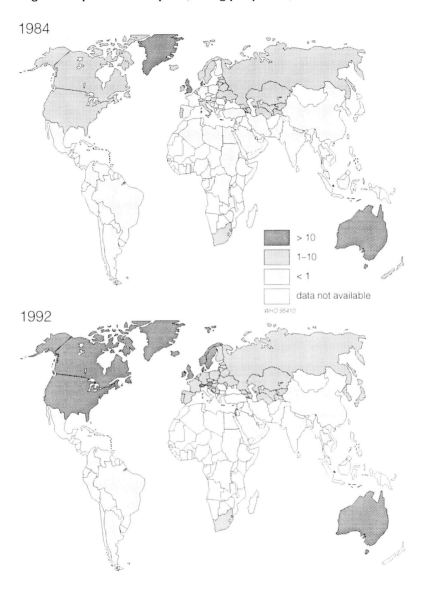

Sources of data: International Narcotics Control Board; United Nations Population and Vital Statistics. Maps reproduced by permission of the WHO Collaborating Center for Symptom Evaluation in Cancer Care, Madison, WI, USA.

unavailability of drugs is often due to a combination of factors, such as inadequate funding of health services, lack of health care delivery infrastructure and inadequate facilities for the storage and distribution of medicines.

These problems are being addressed by WHO through its Action Programme on Essential Drugs. This programme recommends that a national policy on essential drugs should exist in every country, together with an action plan to guarantee the availability at a reasonable cost of a limited number of drugs of significant thera-peutic value. The goal is to satisfy the health care needs of the majority of the population. More than 100 countries have so far adopted lists of essential drugs.

The model list of essential drugs (2) includes three opioid anal-gesics. Codeine and morphine are on the main list; pethidine is on the complementary list. In many countries, however, morphine and other opioids are not available, or available only under very strict conditions, because of national laws aimed at preventing drug abuse. Some of these laws were established long before oral opioids became widely recognized as indispensable for the treat-ment of cancer pain. In such cases, it is essential for health care workers and drug regulators to cooperate in order to make opioid analgesics available while preventing their abuse. The next chapter reviews the Single Convention on Narcotic Drugs, explains the steps that must be taken to make morphine and other opioids available for the treatment of pain, and offers suggestions for doing this efficiently.

The participants in the drug distribution chain

At the outset, it should be emphasized that each participant in the chain of distribution should fulfil all the legal requirements. The chain of distribution includes:

- the national drug regulatory authority
- importers and exporters
- manufacturers
- wholesalers
- doctors, nurses and pharmacists.

The Single Convention on Narcotic Drugs

Description and purpose

The 1961 Single Convention on Narcotic Drugs, as amended by the 1972 Protocol (*6*, *8*), is the principal international treaty regulating availability of opioids. It classifies the opioids, and requires the registration of all handlers and the estimation of medical needs for opioids. It establishes rules concerning production, manufacture and distribution, and requires statistical reports. The Single Convention governs how opioids are shipped between countries, using a system of import and export approval. The treaty also defines to some extent the requirements for safe distribution within a country.

Governments that are party to the Single Convention have agreed to bring their laws and regulations into line with its requirements. A list of the parties is updated and published annually by the INCB (*9*). Countries that are not party to the Single Convention often follow its basic procedures.

The preamble of the Single Convention on Narcotic Drugs (*6*) recognizes that "the medical use of narcotic drugs continues to be indispensable for the relief of pain" [and] "addiction to narcotic drugs constitutes a serious evil".

Thus, the broad purpose of the treaty is to prevent the abuse of narcotics or opioids, while guaranteeing their availability for medical use.

The Single Convention classifies the opioids into four schedules, depending on each drug's dependence potential, abuse liability and therapeutic usefulness. These schedules do not necessarily correspond with those in national laws. The stronger opioid analgesics, such as fentanyl, morphine, hydromorphone and oxycodone are in Schedule I. Codeine and its derivatives, which are less strictly controlled, are in Schedule II. Schedule III contains specified preparations of codeine and dextropropoxyphene that are exempted from certain requirements. Schedule IV contains opioids that are considered to be particularly susceptible to abuse.

Exceptions

Codeine

Preparations containing not more than 100 mg of codeine with one or more other ingredients per dosage unit, and those with a concentration of not more than 2.5% codeine in undivided preparations, such as syrups, are exempted from certain control measures under the Single Convention.

Buprenorphine and pentazocine

These drugs are controlled by the Convention on Psychotropic Substances, 1971.

The drug distribution system

A country obtains its supply of opioids for medical purposes by importing them from another country, manufacturing them itself, or both. These opioids are then distributed by manufacturers or wholesalers to hospitals and pharmacies, and subsequently dispensed to patients by health care personnel.

The Single Convention requires that all individuals and enterprises in the distribution system should be licensed or otherwise appropriately authorized, and that transfers of opioids take place only between properly registered parties. Patients may use opioids only according to a physician's prescription. Certain records must be kept, and reports on consumption must be filed with the national regulatory authority. These, along with security arrangements and inspections, permit the detection of "leakage" or "diversion" from the legitimate system of drug distribution.

National estimates of medical need for opioids

It is vital that a country should have enough opioids to meet the demand for treatment of patients in pain. The INCB has recognized that opioids are underused in the treatment of pain, especially cancer pain, and has called on governments to re-evaluate their needs.

Every year, national drug regulatory authorities prepare an estimate of the amount of Schedule I opioids that will be needed in the country during the following year. The estimate must be submitted to the INCB six months in advance of the period to which it applies. Under the Single Convention, the quantity of opioids manufactured in or imported into a country must not exceed the government's official estimate of the amount needed.

The treaty requires the INCB to confirm the national estimate before the national government may permit the import or manufacture of opioids. In this way, excessive manufacture or import can be monitored and the risk of diversion to non-medical use is minimized.

The treaty also requires the INCB to endeavour to ensure that opioids are available for medical purposes, and to confirm national estimates as quickly as possible. If an annual estimate proves to be inadequate, the national drug regulatory authority is permitted by treaty to submit an amendment to the INCB; the INCB will confirm amendments as soon as possible.

The responsibility for determining the amount of opioids necessary to meet the medical need in a country rests entirely with the national government, in particular with the drug regulatory authority. Countries may use different methods to calculate the estimate, but the INCB must be informed of the method used and of any changes. Typically, an estimate will reflect to some degree the amount of each opioid consumed in previous years.

Communication between health personnel and regulators

Communication between health workers and drug regulators is essential in order to ensure that each understands the other's aims. It is important for pain management experts and medical associations to understand the opioid distribution system in their country, learn about the national estimate of opioid needs, and be aware of the concerns of regulators. Opioid abuse is a reality, and health care workers must cooperate in the campaign to prevent diversion.

It is also important for regulators to learn about the importance of pain relief both for individual patients and for public health in general. Information about cancer pain, where and how cancer patients are treated, and the training of health care personnel will help regulators whose job it is to ensure the integrity of the distribution system. The knowledge that opioid use needs to increase will help regulators to make appropriate changes in the annual estimate.

Health care personnel should make sure that regulators know the salient facts related to pain relief, for example:

- Psychological dependence is rare among cancer patients who receive opioids for pain.

- Oral forms of morphine are preferred because the patient may be able to live at home, and painful injections are eliminated. However, the oral dose needs to be 3–6 times higher than the injected dose to achieve the same degree of pain relief. Thus, the total amount of drug needed will increase significantly; this should be taken into account in preparing the national estimate.

- Pethidine, often relied upon for treatment of acute pain, is not recommended for patients with chronic pain because accumulation of a toxic metabolite may occur, causing myoclonus and seizures. Morphine and other opioids are preferred, and should be included in the national estimate.

Health care workers should tell regulators exactly which opioids are needed, including the dosages and dosage forms required, in order to ensure that the estimate is adequate to meet the needs of patients.

Obtaining a supply of opioids

After the estimate has been confirmed by the INCB, a country may either import or manufacture opioids. In both cases, the participants in the distribution chain should endeavour to ensure that the supply is reliable. Interruptions in the distribution of opioids is distressing for both patients and families and must be avoided.

Domestic manufacture

Some or all of the opioids needed may be manufactured by enterprises in the country itself, which will be regulated (or operated) by the government. Regulation of manufacture of opioid products includes licensing, requirements for record-keeping and reporting, and quality control. Resources are required for record-keeping, to provide secure facilities and maintain security procedures from the acquisition of raw materials until the distribution of the finished products, in order to prevent diversion.

The products available in a country may be limited to the opioids and dosage forms that have been approved for marketing by the national health authority.

A manufacturer may distribute the finished products directly to licensed pharmacies or hospitals, or they may be distributed by a wholesaler. Wholesalers must also be licensed by the national drug regulatory authority, and must obey rules concerning security and record-keeping.

The import/export system

Often, some or all of the opioid products a country needs are imported. The import and export requirements of the Single Convention are outlined here, so that the participants in the opioid distribution system can see what needs to be done to complete the process quickly. Specific requirements may vary from country to country.

The Single Convention lays down a step-by-step process to ensure that the movement of opioids between countries occurs only after authorization by the drug regulatory authorities, and that the amounts imported stay within the approved estimate of the importing country. The import and export certificates are the proof that the products are changing hands legally. Both certificates must be approved and must accompany each shipment. There is no standard certificate, although a model import certificate (Annex 2) has been developed by the United Nations Commission on Narcotic Drugs.

The import certificate
The following information must appear on the import certificate:

- the certificate number,
- the name of the drug,
- the international nonproprietary name (INN) of the drug (*10*),
- the exact description and quantity of the drug, including strength(s) and dosage form(s),
- the name and address of the importer,
- the name and address of the exporter,
- the period of validity of the certificate.

Steps in the import/export process
The import/export process is outlined below and in Fig. 4. It should be noted that many countries also have a certification procedure to prevent marketing of pharmaceutical products that are falsely labelled, counterfeit or substandard (*11*).

1. The entity wishing to import a substance controlled under the Single Convention applies to its regulatory authority for an import certificate.

2. The regulatory authority considers whether the company is properly licensed and whether the drug and amount are within the national estimate; if approved, an original import certificate and one copy are issued.

Fig. 4. Steps in opioid importation

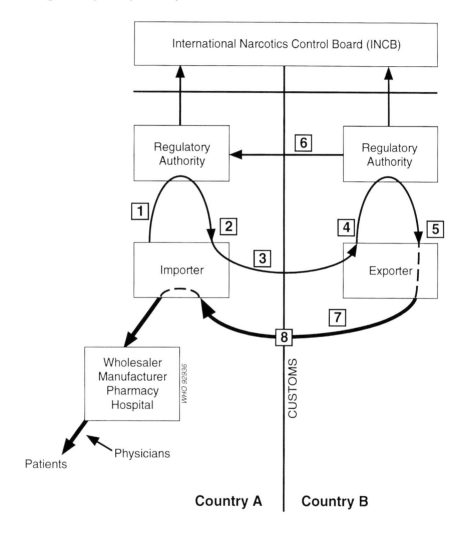

3. The importer sends the original of the import certificate to the entity proposing to export the substance.

4. The exporter applies to its drug regulatory authority for an export certificate.

5. The regulatory authority in the exporting country checks that an import certificate has been issued and that the exporter is properly licensed; if the application is approved, an export certificate is issued.

6. The regulatory authority in the exporting country sends a copy of the export certificate to the regulatory authority in the importing country.

7. The exporter ships the drugs to the importer, along with the originals of the export certificate and import certificate.

8. The shipment must pass a customs inspection.

9. The importer sends both certificates to its regulatory authority.

It is important that there is complete, accurate and prompt communication between the participants to minimize the time between the various steps in the process.

The reporting system

National drug regulatory authorities must report all imports and exports of opioids to the INCB every quarter. They are also required to make an annual inventory and report the total amount of opioids manufactured, consumed and in stock. The annual inventory does not include drugs stored in pharmacies, which for official purposes are considered to have been consumed.

The INCB, in turn, uses these data to prepare reports and monitor global production and consumption of opioids. INCB statistical reports (9) can be useful to health care workers who need to know the quantity of opioids consumed in their country in previous years. These statistics also provide a global picture of morphine consumption. For statistical purposes, a "defined daily dose" (DDD) has been calculated to allow a rough comparison of consumption of drugs of different potencies in different countries. The DDD for morphine is 30 mg. It must be emphasized that the DDD has no significance in terms of medical use or for drawing up estimates of opioid needs, but is intended only as a tool for analysing differences in consumption around the world.

The annual reports of the INCB provide useful information about its work, as well as patterns of medical use and diversion of opioids. The INCB also produces periodic special reports that focus attention on critical issues, such as the 1989 special report *Demand for and supply of opiates for medical and scientific needs* (*12*) which called on governments to re-evaluate medical needs for opioids.

Is the international system working?

In recent years, the INCB has reported to the United Nations Economic and Social Council that the international control system continues to operate satisfactorily (*13*).

> Diversion of narcotic drugs from the licit trade into illicit channels remains relatively rare and the quantities involved are small in comparison with the large volume of transactions. That holds true for drugs in the international trade as well as in domestic wholesale circuits.

The INCB has also reported on its efforts to improve opioid availability for the treatment of pain. In the special report mentioned above (*12*), the INCB reviewed the availability of opioids for medical and scientific purposes in consultation with WHO. The INCB concluded that the medical need for opioids is not being fully met, particularly in respect of cancer pain. The INCB made recommendations to governments, WHO, professional associations and medical instructors, on the need to:

- improve methods of assessing medical needs;
- develop a monitoring system to show whether medical needs for opioids are being met and to indicate corrective actions required;
- identify obstacles to the appropriate use of opioids and facilitate their availability in cases of severe pain;
- establish national policies and guidelines on the appropriate medical use of opioids;

- ensure that health professionals are adequately trained in opioid use and informed about drug dependence;

- urge medical instructors and professional medical associations to promote the rational use of opiates for medical purposes while taking measures to ensure that they are not abused.

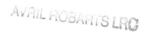

Regulation of health care workers

The Single Convention recognizes that individual governments must decide the level of regulation of the individuals directly involved in dispensing opioids — pharmacists, physicians and nurses. However, it expresses several principles that should be observed:

- individuals must be authorized to dispense opioids by their professional licence to practise, or be specially licensed to do so;

- movement of opioids may occur only between duly authorized parties;

- a medical prescription is required before opioids may be dispensed to a patient.

Drug abuse versus patient need

The Single Convention recognizes that governments have the right to impose further restrictions if they consider it necessary, to prevent diversion and misuse of opioids. However, this right must be continually balanced against the responsibility to ensure opioid availability for medical purposes.

In deciding the appropriate level of regulation, governments should bear in mind the dual aims of the Single Convention. The INCB has observed that in some countries fear of drug abuse has resulted in laws and regulations, or interpretations thereof, that make it unnecessarily difficult to obtain opioids for medical use.

> Prevention of availability of opiates for medical use does not necessarily guarantee prevention of the abuse of illicitly procured opiates. Overly restrictive approaches may, in the end, merely result in depriving a majority of the population of access to opiate medications (*12*).

The WHO Expert Committee on Cancer Pain Relief and Active Supportive Care (7) has commented on special multiple-copy prescription programmes that are required by governments in some countries and in several states of the United States of America. Typically, these programmes reduce prescribing of covered drugs by 50% or more. Although the Expert Committee acknowledged that they may reduce careless prescribing and "multiple doctoring", it also noted:

> . . . the extent to which these programmes restrict or inhibit the prescribing of opioids to patients who need them should also be questioned.

Health care workers may be reluctant to prescribe, stock or dispense opioids if they feel that there is a possibility of their professional licences being suspended or revoked by the governing authority in cases where large quantities of opioids are provided to an individual, even though the medical need for such drugs can be proved.

Suggested guidelines for regulation of health professionals

It is understood that regulatory requirements for physicians, nurses and pharmacists to dispense opioids to patients will differ from country to country. However, the following are general criteria that can be used to develop a practical system.

1. *Legal authority.* Physicians, nurses and pharmacists should be legally empowered to prescribe, dispense and administer opioids to patients in accordance with local needs.

2. *Accountability.* They must dispense opioids for medical purposes only and must be held responsible in law if they dispense them for non-medical purposes.

   Appropriate records must be kept. If physicians are required to keep records other than those associated with good medical practice, the extra work incurred should be practicable and should not impede medical activities. Hospitals and pharmacists must be legally responsible for safe storage and the recording of opioids received and dispensed.

Reasonable record-keeping and accountability provisions should not discourage health care workers from prescribing or stocking adequate supplies of opioids.

3. *Prescriptions.* A prescription for opioids should contain at least the following information:

- name and address of the patient,
- date of issue,
- drug name, dosage strength and form, quantity prescribed,
- directions for use,
- physician's name and business address,
- physician's signature.

4. *Patient access.* Opioids should be available in locations that will be accessible to as many cancer patients as possible.

5. *Medical decisions.* Decisions concerning the type of drug to be used, the amount of the prescription and the duration of therapy are best made by medical professionals on the basis of the individual needs of each patient, and not by regulation.

6. *Dependence.* Physical dependence, which may develop when opioids are used to treat chronic pain, should not be confused with psychological dependence.

References

1. Foley KM, Arbit E. Management of cancer pain. In: DeVita V Jr et al., ed. *Cancer — principles and practice of oncology*, 3rd ed. Philadelphia, Lippincott, 1989: pp. 2064–2087.

2. *The use of essential drugs: sixth report of the WHO Expert Committee.* Geneva, World Health Organization, 1995 (WHO Technical Report Series, No. 850).

3. *WHO Expert Committee on Drug Dependence: twenty-eighth report.* Geneva, World Health Organization, 1993 (WHO Technical Report Series, No. 836).

4. Inturrisi CE. Management of cancer pain: pharmacology and principles of management. *Cancer*, 1989, 63:2308–2320.

5. Twycross RG. *Therapeutics in terminal cancer*, 3rd ed. Oxford, Radcliffe Medical Press, 1995.

6. *Single Convention on Narcotic Drugs, 1961 (as amended by the 1972 Protocol).* New York, United Nations, 1977.

7. *Cancer pain relief and palliative care: report of a WHO Expert Committee.* Geneva, World Health Organization, 1990 (WHO Technical Report Series, No. 804).

8. *Commentary on the Single Convention on Narcotic Drugs, 1961.* New York, United Nations, 1973.

9. International Narcotics Control Board. *Narcotic drugs: estimated world requirements for 1992; statistics for 1990.* New York, United Nations, 1991.

10. *International nonproprietary names (INN) for pharmaceutical substances; cumulative list No. 8.* Geneva, World Health Organization, 1992.

11. *WHO Expert Committee on Specifications for Pharmaceutical Preparations: thirty-first report.* Geneva, World Health Organization, 1990 (WHO Technical Report Series, No. 790).

12. International Narcotics Control Board. *Demand for and supply of opiates for medical and scientific needs.* New York, United Nations, 1989.

13. International Narcotics Control Board. *Report of the International Narcotics Control Board for 1990.* New York, United Nations, 1990.

14. *National cancer control programmes: policies and managerial guidelines.* Geneva World Health Organization, 1995.

Selected further reading

Doyle D, Hanks GWC, Macdonald N, eds. *Oxford textbook of palliative medicine*. Oxford, Oxford University Press, 1993.

Foley KM, Bonica JJ, Ventafridda, V, eds. *Second International Congress on Cancer Pain*. New York, Raven Press, 1990 (Advances in Pain Research and Therapy, Vol. 16).

Twycross RG. *Pain relief in advanced cancer*. Edinburgh, Churchill Livingstone, 1994.

US Department of Health and Human Services. *Management of cancer pain*. Rockville, MD, 1994 (Clinical Practice Guideline, No. 9).

Use of terms

Narcotic   In this publication, the term "narcotic" is used only in relation to the Single Convention on Narcotic Drugs, 1961, in which the term is used in a legal rather than a pharmacological sense. The Single Convention includes substances that are not narcotics from a pharmacological point of view, for example marijuana and cocaine.

Opioid   In this publication, opioid refers to codeine, morphine, and other natural and synthetic drugs whose effects are mediated by specific receptors in the central and peripheral nervous systems.

Tolerance   Increased resistance to the usual effects of a drug as a result of long-term continual use.

Physical dependence   "Physical dependence" is used to describe the neuroadaptation of the body to the presence of an opioid, and is characterized by the onset of acute symptoms and signs of withdrawal if the opioid is stopped or an opioid antagonist is administered.

Psychological dependence   "Psychological dependence" is used to describe a behavioural pattern characterized by a craving for the mood-altering effects of a drug and an overwhelming preoccupation with obtaining and using the drug.

ANNEX 2

Model import certificate

MODEL FORM OF IMPORT CERTIFICATE
Certificate of Official Approval of Import No. . . . .   (date) . . . .

INTERNATIONAL OPIUM CONVENTION OF 1925
SINGLE CONVENTION ON NARCOTIC DRUGS, 1961

1. To be completed in all cases

1. I hereby certify that [name of Authority]. . . . . , being the Authority charged with the administration of the law relating to the drugs to which the 1925 and 1961 Conventions apply, has approved the importation by

(a) Name, address and business of importer

(a) . . . .
. . . .
. . . .

(b) Exact description and amount of drugs to be imported, including the international nonproprietary name, if any.

of (b) . . . .
. . . .
. . . .
. . . .
. . . .

(c) Name and address of firm in exporting country from which the drug is to be obtained.

from (c) . . . .
. . . .
. . . .
subject to the following conditions:

(d) State any special conditions to be observed, e.g. not to be imported through the post.

(d) . . . .
. . . .
. . . .

2. To be completed only if the consignment is required for other than medical or scientific purposes.

2. See note below.

3. Duration of validity

3. . . . .
Signed on behalf of [name of Authority]
. . . .
Signature . . . .
Official rank. . . . .
Date. . . . .

Note: It should be indicated for which of the following purposes the consignment to be imported is required:

(a) for the preparation of a flavouring agent in the case of coca leaves;
(b) for legitimate purposes in the case of poppy straw;
(c) (i) for smoking in the case of opium; (ii) for quasi-medical and non-medical purposes other than smoking in the case of opium; (iii) for chewing in the case of coca leaves; (iv) for non-medical purposes in the case of cannabis, cannabis resin, extracts and tinctures of cannabis and their preparations (Article 49 of the 1961 Convention).